Would you like to stop your excessive sweating but don't know how?

Have you tried many things but nothing has ever really worked?

Then read this practical stop sweating guide and discover...

What can cause excessive sweating?

What is the main cause of excessive sweating?

Is excessive sweating a sign of cancer?

How do you stop sweating so much?

Can Sweating be a sign of cancer?

What is excessive sweating a sign of?

What can cause sudden sweating?

What is the reason for sweating?

What causes excessive body sweating?

Is sweating a sign of a heart attack?

What is excessive sweating a sign of?

Is there a pill to stop excessive sweating?

How can I stop excessive sweating?

Is excessive sweating a sign of diabetes?

How can I stop excessive sweating naturally?

Did you know that excessive sweating in the armpits, feet and hands is called "hyperhidrosis"? Do you suffer it, especially when summer arrives? So, you can not miss this note where we will tell you what are the best natural remedies for excessive sweating. Pay close attention and say goodbye to the abundant perspiration that makes you ashamed!

What is sweat for?

As a first step, we have to understand what the purpose of sweating is: to regulate body temperature. When the skin is more degrees than normal, the body begins to perspire to cool it. That is why we sweat when we are very warm, when we enter a room with too high heating, when we have a fever, when we are in the sun, when the ambient temperature exceeds 30 ° C or when we play sports.

Diabetes: it can produce a profuse and excessive sweating when hypoglycemia occurs, that is, when the sugar goes down. This happens many times because of excess insulin.

Cancer: hidden cancers, which can produce very vague symptoms and are not usually identified, often come with profuse sweating, which is a clue for the doctor to diagnose the disease.

Why do I sweat a lot?

It is one of the questions I receive the most and the answers can be many.

But in most cases an excess of sweat has to do with stressful situations and / or anxiety.

"I Don't Have Excessive Sweating Anymore"

My sweating kept getting worse and my doctor told me the only option was surgery. Then I found a simple natural remedy and in just a few weeks my excessive sweating was gone.

==> Here Is What I'm Doing...

Unless you have night sweats, chances are that the reasons why you are wetting your armpits or are seeing an excess of sweat in your body have to do with an imbalance in your nervous system.

Prevention

The main prevention measures are:

Use fresh clothes that allow perspiration and preferably synthetic fibers instead of natural fibers, as they repel sweat and keep clothes dry.

Keep the home and workplace cool and well ventilated.

Avoid the consumption of alcohol, coffee, tea, tobacco and spicy foods that can stimulate the production of sweat.

Reduce the psychological effects related to sweating, such as stress, tension and anxiety.

Primary hyperhidrosis often manifests in childhood, progressively getting worse in the pubertal period, and then decreases again in old age. Its genetic component is very important, and the frequently affected areas are the palms of the hands, the soles of the feet and the armpits. They can also sweat excessively on the face, scalp, inframammary area or groins, although there are fewer cases.

There is a second type of hyperhidrosis, secondary, that can appear at any age. Usually a symptom that you suffer from another disease or hormonal disorder, such as: anxiety or depression, hyperthyroidism, obesity, menopause, and even due to taking some drugs that act on the nervous system.

Antiperspirants

They are substances that we apply directly to the skin to reduce excess sweating. Its effectiveness is scientifically recognized and highlights the role of aluminum chloride for its ability to plug eccrine glands and de-structure keratin. They should be used at night and with dry skin.

The moment we notice the clinical improvement we should space its use 2-3 times a week. Its main adverse effect is skin irritation, which may limit its use. On the other hand, there is no evidence that aluminum can cause mutation or DNA damage that can cause cancer.

When does excessive sweat appear for the first time?

The way in which this problem occurs in a usual way, is making its appearance in childhood or early adolescence and remains in time until adulthood, in some people (less than 10%) it diminishes or disappears when the person is an adult.

"I Don't Have Excessive Sweating Anymore"

My sweating kept getting worse and my doctor told me the only option was surgery. Then I found a simple natural remedy and in just a few weeks my excessive sweating was gone.

==> Here Is What I'm Doing...

Beware of deodorant. Do not use scented deodorant if your sweat smells. In the end, the mixture between the smell of sweat and that of the product that we throw away is more unpleasant than the smell that we suffer.

The best thing, deodorants in bar and that are transparent so as not to stain the clothes, and always after washing and drying well.

When there is an excess of sweating in the feet, the development of the bacteria is favored, giving rise to problems and discomforts that affect us in our daily life:

Bad smell of feet and shoes

Sensation of discomfort from wet feet

Bacterial infections

Rashes

Mushrooms in ones and feet

Medications: in case the pathology is of a higher level, it is recommended to use anticholinergics to prevent the stimulation of the sweat glands, but it is important to consult the doctor before making any decision, since its side effects include dizziness and problems when urinating .

Iontophoresis: consists of closing by electricity and temporarily the sweat gland. It is used to a greater extent to treat excessive sweating of hands and feet. Although there are no very common side effects, blisters may occur.

In recent years, a new medical treatment has been introduced consisting of the use of botulinum toxin type A which has proven to be a safe and effective treatment for primary and hand axillary hyperhidrosis, with high levels of patient satisfaction.

The technique involves the subcutaneous injection of the toxin into the corresponding hyperhidrosis area, which causes a blockage of the nerve endings responsible for the sweat glands.

The effects, that is to say, the reduction in sweating, begin to be noticed between 2 and 4 days and the symptoms remit in a week, but unfortunately they can reappear after about 3 months in the case of hands and up to 8 months after in axillary hyperhidrosis.

Prevention and treatment of excess sweat

Hyperhidrosis is chronic, but we can take some measures to prevent excess sweating. From the outset, it is advisable to change the deodorant for an antiperspirant that controls and reduces abundant sweating, applying it before going to sleep to benefit from its effect the next day.

It will also help us to avoid tight clothing and choose clothes from natural fabrics such as cotton, silk or linen. If we are going to spend a lot of time outside, wearing spare clothes will make us feel more comfortable and safe.